HERBAL REMEDIES FOR EPI

Harnessing Herbal Solutions For Optimal Digestive Health, Holistic Healing, Sustainable Well-Being And Balancing Digestive Function

DR. CARDEN KYRIE

DISCLAIMER

The only goal of this book is informational. Every effort has been taken by the author and publisher to ensure that the information provided is accurate. But the material in this book is given "as is," without any express or implied representation, warranty, or condition as to its accuracy, completeness, or suitability for any particular purpose.

Any loss, damage, or injury resulting from using the information in this book, or from any action or decision made as a result of such use, will not be covered by the author's or publisher's liability. It is recommended that readers seek the assistance of a certified specialist for guidance specific to their situation.

The opinions and viewpoints conveyed in this book belong to the author and may not necessarily represent the official stance or policies of any specified organizations or people. Any likeness to real-life occurrences, places, or people—living or deceased—is wholly coincidental.

No specific product, service, or therapy discussed in this book is endorsed by the author or publisher. Any reference to goods or services is made only for informative reasons and is not intended as a recommendation or endorsement.

Before making any judgments or acting on any information, readers are urged to independently confirm it all. Any unfavorable effects or repercussions arising from the usage of the material included in this book are disclaimed by the author and publisher.

By using this book, you consent to absolving the publisher and author of any and all claims, obligations, or losses resulting from your use of the material in it.

I appreciate your cooperation and understanding.

TABLE OF CONTENTS

CHAPTER ONE

INTRODUCTION TO EPI

EXOCRINE PANCREATIC INSUFFICIENCY (EPI) BACKGROUND

A medical disorder known as exocrine pancreatic insufficiency (EPI) is defined as the pancreas producing or secreting insufficient amounts of digesting enzymes. Because it produces the enzymes amylase, lipase, and protease—which are necessary for the digestion of carbohydrates, lipids, and proteins, respectively—the pancreas plays a critical part in the digestive process. These enzymes are lacking in people with EPI, which causes malabsorption of nutrients and consequent digestive problems.

EPI can have a variety of underlying causes, such as pancreatic surgery, cystic fibrosis, chronic pancreatitis, and certain gastrointestinal problems. Pancreatic tissue may be destroyed as a result of persistent pancreatic inflammation, as observed in chronic pancreatitis, which would hinder the pancreas's capacity to efficiently generate and release enzymes. The hereditary condition known as cystic fibrosis, which affects the creation of thick, sticky mucus that can obstruct the pancreatic ducts and prevent enzymes from passing through, can also be a factor in epilepsy.

EPI can cause weight loss, diarrhea, malnourishment, and discomfort in the abdomen. These symptoms are frequently mild. A combination of clinical assessment, imaging examinations, and laboratory testing, such as fecal elastase and direct pancreatic function tests, are usually used to make the diagnosis. The two main approaches to managing EPI are treating the underlying cause and using medicine to replenish the lacking enzymes.

SYNOPSIS OF HERBAL TREATMENTS

With a long history of usage in treating a wide range of medical ailments, herbal remedies have been a crucial component of traditional medical systems throughout the world for ages. These treatments take advantage of the healing qualities of natural substances by using plants and plant extracts as their source. Exploring the possibility of herbal medicines as a complement to traditional medical approaches for a variety of disorders has gained more attention in recent years.

Herbal medicines are popular because they are regarded as safer than synthetic pharmaceuticals, can be easily obtained, and frequently have a lesser potential for side effects. Numerous plants include anti-inflammatory, antioxidant, and antibacterial bioactive chemicals in them, which makes them appealing options for promoting health and well-being. It is imperative to acknowledge that the effectiveness of herbal remedies is subject to variation, and their utilization must be done cautiously, especially when dealing with particular medical disorders.

Regarding digestive health, several herbs are thought to have qualities that could facilitate digestion and lessen symptoms related to illnesses such as exocrine pancreatic insufficiency. For example, several herbal medicines are believed to contain anti-inflammatory properties that may help reduce the inflammation linked to chronic pancreatitis, which is a prevalent cause of end-stage pancreatitis. Those who are thinking about using herbal medicines should speak with medical specialists to make sure these complementary therapies are safe, don't conflict with prescription drugs, and don't make pre-existing conditions worse.

CHAPTER TWO

A COMPREHENSIVE OVERVIEW OF EXOCRINE PANCREATIC INSUFFICIENCY (EPI)

EPI: WHAT IS IT?

The disease known as exocrine pancreatic insufficiency (EPI) is characterized by the pancreas's incapacity to generate and secrete an adequate quantity of digestive enzymes into the small intestine. These digestive enzymes, which include lipase, amylase, and protease, are essential for metabolizing proteins, lipids, and carbohydrates found in meals. Malabsorption occurs when the pancreas is unable to produce enough of these enzymes, which prevents the body from correctly absorbing vital nutrients.

REASONS AND DANGER FACTORS

The etiology of exocrine pancreatic insufficiency is frequently linked to illnesses affecting the pancreas. Among the frequent offenders are pancreatic cancer, cystic fibrosis, chronic pancreatitis, and some gastrointestinal procedures. Repeated pancreatic inflammation in chronic pancreatitis can harm glandular tissue and reduce the generation of enzymes. Furthermore, diseases like cystic fibrosis can alter the makeup of pancreatic secretions, which can affect how well the digestive enzymes work.

A genetic predisposition, certain autoimmune illnesses, and a history of pancreatic problems are among the risk factors that lead to the development of EPI. Pancreatic dysfunction and diabetes frequently occur, and this can increase the risk of EPI. Lifestyle choices like smoking and binge drinking can increase a person's chance of developing pancreatic disorders and increase their susceptibility to exocrine pancreatic insufficiency.

SIGNS AND PROGNOSIS

Exocrine pancreatic insufficiency frequently has nonspecific symptoms, which makes an early diagnosis difficult. Diarrhea, weight loss, discomfort in the abdomen, and malnutrition as a result of nutrient malabsorption are typical symptoms. In addition, bloating, gas, and foul-smelling stools—all signs of undigested fat—may be experienced by people with EPI.

Several diagnostics, clinical assessments, and medical history are used in the diagnosis of EPI. The fecal elastase-1 test is frequently used to assess the pancreatic enzyme elastase. Imaging tests that include endoscopic ultrasonography, magnetic resonance imaging (MRI), and computed tomography (CT) scans can help detect structural anomalies in the pancreas. Testing for nutritional deficits linked to malabsorption can be done with blood testing.

TRADITIONAL THERAPY CHOICES

The mainstay of care for patients with exocrine pancreatic insufficiency is enzyme replacement therapy (ERT). To help with digestion, pancreatic enzyme supplements containing lipase, amylase, and protease are given with meals. By supporting the appropriate breakdown and absorption of nutrients, these supplements aid in making up for insufficient pancreatic enzymes.

Dietary changes and enzyme replacement are essential for the management of epilepsy. To combat malnutrition, a low-fat diet, frequent short meals, and nutritional supplements could be advised. An essential component of the overall treatment plan is taking care of the underlying problem, such as treating cystic fibrosis or chronic pancreatitis.

Additional measures can be required in severe cases if problems like diabetes or nutritional deficits occur. To guarantee the best possible management of exocrine pancreatic insufficiency and to customize treatment programs to each patient's needs, close monitoring and cooperation with healthcare providers are crucial.

CHAPTER THREE

HERBS' FUNCTION IN EPI MANAGEMENT
OVERVIEW OF HERBAL MEDICINE

For millennia, herbal medicine has been an essential component of traditional healing methods in many different cultures, providing a natural approach to health and well-being. Herbal therapy for Exocrine Pancreatic Insufficiency (EPI) is an example of a holistic approach to medicine that recognizes the interdependence of all body systems.

Herbal treatments are recognized for their wide range of medicinal benefits and are derived from plant sources. Herbs are quite important when it comes to managing epilepsy in the context of maintaining digestive health and reducing pancreatic insufficiency symptoms.

HOW HERBS HELP PROMOTE HEALTHY DIGESTIVE SYSTEM

The digestive system is an intricate web of organs that cooperate to process food and absorb it. Herbs support digestive health via a variety of methods. Some herbs have a carminative quality that might help reduce bloating and stomach symptoms. For instance, ginger and peppermint have long been used to ease digestive issues and alleviate pain related to decrease pancreatic function.

Furthermore, some herbs increase the production of digestive enzymes, which is important when considering EPI because pancreatic enzymes are deficient in the condition. Herbs that aid in the breakdown of lipids, proteins, and carbs include dandelion root, turmeric, and fennel. These herbs may also increase the synthesis of digestive enzymes. For those with EPI, this enzymatic assistance might be quite important as it improves overall digestive efficiency and nutritional absorption.

Additionally, herbs support the general well-being of the lining of the stomach. For example, marshmallow roots and slippery elm are recognized for their mucilaginous qualities, which coat the mucous membranes of the digestive tract in a protective layer. Those with EPI who can have gastrointestinal pain can find relief from inflammation and irritation because of this protective barrier.

SECURITY AND POINTS TO REMEMBER

Even though herbal medicines can be a great help in managing EPI, it's important to utilize them carefully and under a doctor's supervision. Not every person can use all herbs, and it's important to carefully examine any potential conflicts with prescription drugs or pre-existing medical issues.

Herbal remedies must be standardized to guarantee constant potency and effectiveness. Herbal supplements should be prescribed in a way that best suits the needs of the individual, taking into consideration aspects like age, general health, and the intensity of symptoms associated with encephalitis.

It's also critical to be informed of any possible adverse reactions and side effects linked to specific herbs. Herbal treatments must be safely and effectively integrated into the overall management of encephalitis (EPI) by being closely monitored for side effects and promptly communicating with a healthcare provider in case of any concerns.

Let's sum up by saying that herbs have a variety of functions in the management of endoplasmic reticulum, including mucosal protection, enzyme stimulation, and digestive assistance. Herbal medication offers a safe and effective natural solution for treating EPI symptoms, but in each situation, a careful and knowledgeable approach is required to assure safety and efficacy. It is possible to improve the quality of life for people with EPI by incorporating herbs into a thorough treatment plan under the guidance of medical professionals.

CHAPTER FOUR

HERBS TO HELP WITH DIGESTION
MINT PEPPER

Long acknowledged for its many health advantages, peppermint is especially beneficial for digestive health. Menthol, one of the main ingredients in peppermint, is well-known for its calming and soothing effects on the digestive system. Many digestive problems can be helped by peppermint, and it can also help with disorders like exocrine pancreatic insufficiency (EPI).

The insufficient synthesis or secretion of digesting enzymes by the pancreas is the hallmark of exocrine pancreatic insufficiency. In the digestive tract, these enzymes are essential for the breakdown of proteins, lipids, and carbohydrates. It has been determined that peppermint is a natural medicine that could provide relief for those with EPI.

ADVANTAGES OF EPI

The ability of peppermint to relax gastrointestinal tract muscles, particularly the sphincter of Oddi, a muscular valve that regulates the passage of digestive juices from the pancreas and gallbladder, is beneficial for endoplasmic reticulum (EPI). Peppermint may help with the release of digestive enzymes and improve the process of digestion for those with epilepsy by encouraging muscle relaxation.

There are several methods for incorporating peppermint into a routine for controlling EPI. A widely used approach is the ingestion of peppermint tea. Adding peppermint to one's everyday diet can be calming and delightful, and peppermint tea is widely accessible. The warm beverage might also aid in calming the digestive tract and easing EPI-related discomfort.

PEPPERMINT: HOW TO USE IT FOR EPI

Using peppermint oil is a useful approach to take advantage of peppermint's benefits for EPI. Because peppermint oil supplements come in pill form, people can easily incorporate them into their routine. Before beginning any new supplementation, it is imperative to speak with a healthcare provider, particularly for individuals who are already on medication or have pre-existing health conditions.

For those who would rather take a culinary approach, fresh peppermint leaves can be a garnish for a variety of foods or added to salads and smoothies. This not only brings a taste explosion but also integrates peppermint's natural digestive benefits into the diet.

Among the many beneficial herbs for supporting digestive health, peppermint is particularly beneficial for those with inflammatory bowel syndrome (EPI). The natural qualities of peppermint, whether sipped as a tea, taken as a supplement, or mixed into food, can help persons with this illness have a more pleasant digestive system. As with any herbal therapy, it's important to speak with a medical practitioner to figure out how best to incorporate peppermint into a person's overall health regimen.

DIGESTIVE HEALTH BENEFITS OF GINGER:

For generations, people have valued the therapeutic benefits of ginger, which comes from the root of the Zingiber officinale plant, especially for their ability to support digestive health.

Gingerol is a bioactive molecule with anti-inflammatory and antioxidant properties that is one of the main ingredients of ginger. Because of these qualities, ginger is a great ally for treating a wide range of digestive problems, from nausea to more complicated ailments like exocrine pancreatic insufficiency (EPI).

ADVANTAGES OF EPI

A disorder known as exocrine pancreatic insufficiency occurs when the pancreas is unable to generate enough enzymes for adequate meal digestion. Because ginger stimulates the synthesis of digestive enzymes, it has demonstrated promising advantages for those with EPI. Ginger's active ingredients, especially gingerol, help break down proteins and lipids to make digestion easier. Furthermore, the anti-inflammatory qualities of ginger might aid in reducing the inflammation linked to EPI, improving overall digestive comfort.

According to research, ginger may increase the activity of pancreatic enzymes, which will help with nutrient absorption and digestion. This is important since malabsorption of vital minerals is a common problem for people with EPI. People with inflammatory bowel disease (EPI) may benefit from adding ginger to their regimen since it can help with better nutrient absorption, less discomfort, and better digestion.

GINGER'S USE FOR EPI

Ginger can be added to food in a variety of ways to maximize its advantages for people with epilepsy. A popular approach is the use of ginger tea. Grate fresh ginger root and steep it in boiling water to make ginger tea. This makes it possible for the active ingredients to seep into the water, producing a calming and gastrointestinal-friendly drink. To get the most out of this tea's digestive benefits, it is best to drink it either before or after meals.

Ginger can be added to food in a variety of ways, not only tea. You may add freshly grated or minced ginger to stir-fries, soups, stews, and even smoothies. Ginger's adaptability allows it to be used in a wide variety of recipes, adding taste and digestive advantages.

Supplements are available for people who want a more concentrated version of ginger. These supplements, which are usually in the form of extracts or capsules, offer a practical approach to including ginger in everyday routines. But before adding supplements to one's regimen, it's imperative to speak with a healthcare provider, particularly for people who are taking medication or have pre-existing health conditions.

Among the many effective natural remedies for supporting digestive health, ginger is especially noteworthy when used in conjunction with exocrine pancreatic insufficiency. Its many advantages, which include enzyme stimulation and anti-inflammatory properties, make it a flexible and affordable choice for anyone looking to improve their digestive health. Whether taken as a supplement, added to food, or drank as tea, ginger provides a comprehensive method of promoting healthy digestion and general well-being.

TURMERIC

The medicinal qualities of turmeric, which is derived from the Curcuma longa plant, have been known for millennia. Turmeric is well known for its numerous health advantages, one of which is its favorable impact on digestive health. Curcumin, a bioactive substance with strong anti-inflammatory and antioxidant qualities, is one of the main ingredients of turmeric. Turmeric has the potential to treat several digestive disorders, including exocrine pancreatic insufficiency (EPI), thanks to these qualities.

EPI is a disorder marked by the pancreas's insufficient production and secretion of digestive enzymes, which makes it difficult for the body to process and absorb nutrients from food. Due in large part to its anti-inflammatory qualities, turmeric has been researched for its potential advantages in treating EPI. EPI may be exacerbated by pancreatic inflammation, and turmeric's anti-inflammatory properties may help ease the illness's symptoms.

ADVANTAGES OF EPI

It has been demonstrated that curcumin, the active component of turmeric, modifies inflammatory pathways and prevents the release of cytokines that promote inflammation. Turmeric may therefore help to lessen pancreatic inflammation, which may enhance the organ's performance and facilitate food digestion.

Turmeric may help digestive health in addition to its anti-inflammatory properties by encouraging the generation of bile. The small intestine's ability to break down and absorb lipids depends on bile. According to some research, turmeric may increase the production of bile, which can help with nutrient absorption and fat breakdown, addressing one of the problems that people with EPI encounter.

HOW TO APPLY GINGER TO EPI

Turmeric can be included in the EPI diet in several ways. Cooking using turmeric as a spice is one popular technique. In addition to adding taste to a range of foods, including stir-fries, soups, and curries, turmeric may provide significant digestive advantages. It is noteworthy that black pepper, which includes piperine, an ingredient that increases curcumin bioavailability, can promote the absorption of curcumin, the active ingredient in turmeric.

Turmeric pills are also available for people who want to take advantage of the benefits of turmeric more directly. When compared to consuming turmeric as a spice, these supplements—which frequently contain a concentrated form of the herb—may offer a more standardized and effective dosage. Before adding supplements to one's regimen, it is best to speak with a healthcare provider, especially if one is taking medication or has pre-existing health issues.

Turmeric has potential as a homeopathic treatment for improving digestive health, especially when used in conjunction with EPI. It is a beneficial supplement to a balanced diet because of its anti-inflammatory qualities and capacity to increase bile production. Adding turmeric to one's diet may help with digestion, whether it is taken as a supplement or used as a spice in cooking.

CHAPTER FIVE

HERBS TO ASSIST THE PANCREAS

THISTLE OF MILK

The herb milk thistle, scientifically named Silybum marianum, has been acknowledged for its possible advantages in promoting pancreatic health. A flavonoid with anti-inflammatory and antioxidant qualities, silymarin is one of the main active ingredients in milk thistle. These characteristics support its capacity to enhance liver function generally, which is strongly associated with pancreatic health.

Milk thistle has drawn interest as a pancreatic support herb due to its ability to lessen oxidative stress-related damage. The pancreas' high metabolic activity and exposure to free radicals make it especially susceptible to oxidative stress. Milk thistle silymarin assists in scavenging these free radicals, lessening the oxidative stress on the pancreas.

Moreover, research has been conducted on milk thistle's potential to treat pancreatic conditions, such as exocrine pancreatic insufficiency (EPI). The condition known as EPI is defined by the pancreas producing and secreting insufficient amounts of digestive enzymes. These enzymes are necessary for the digestive system to properly break down and absorb nutrients.

ADVANTAGES FOR HEPATIC FUNCTION

The anti-inflammatory properties of milk thistle are thought to contribute to the benefits it offers for pancreatic health by perhaps reducing pancreatic inflammation. Since several pancreatic problems are associated with chronic inflammation, milk thistle may improve pancreatic health generally by reducing inflammation.

HOW MILK THISTLE IS USED FOR EPILEPSY

It is worthwhile to investigate the use of milk thistle as a supplemental strategy in the context of EPI. Because of their low synthesis of pancreatic enzymes, people with epilepsy frequently have difficulties with fat and fat-soluble vitamin digestion. By promoting liver function, milk thistle may help improve the way fat is absorbed. This can have an impact on the type and amount of digestive enzymes the pancreas produces.

Milk thistle can be used in a wellness regimen in several ways to support the pancreas, such as tinctures, teas, or supplements. Before beginning any new supplement regimen, though, it's imperative to speak with a healthcare provider, especially if you have any underlying medical concerns or are taking other medications.

In the context of EPI, milk thistle shows great promise as a herb for pancreatic support. Its potential to improve liver function and anti-inflammatory and antioxidant qualities add to its overall benefits for pancreas health. Like any herbal medication, it's crucial to use it carefully and under a doctor's supervision to be sure it's suitable for your particular set of health needs.

DANDELION

Scientifically named Taraxacum officinale, dandelion is a multipurpose herb with a long history of usage in medicine. The potential advantages and therapeutic characteristics of dandelion have drawn attention in the context of pancreatic support. The plant is a helpful addition to dietary regimens targeted at maintaining pancreatic health because it is rich in iron, potassium, calcium, and vitamins A, C, and K.

ADVANTAGES FOR HEPATIC FUNCTION

The capacity of dandelion to promote overall gastrointestinal function and stimulate digestion is one of the plant's main advantages for pancreatic health. It is especially pertinent when discussing Exocrine Pancreatic Insufficiency (EPI), a disorder in which the pancreas is unable to generate enough amounts of digesting enzymes. The ability of dandelion to stimulate the formation of bile, which facilitates the breakdown and assimilation of lipids and fat-soluble vitamins, has been acknowledged. For those with EPI, who frequently experience difficulties absorbing nutrients, this is essential.

Dandelion is also well-known for having anti-inflammatory qualities. Pancreatic diseases are frequently linked to chronic inflammation, and the chemicals in dandelion may be able to reduce pancreatic inflammation. This anti-inflammatory action may lessen some of the symptoms linked to pancreatic problems and help to create an environment that is supportive of pancreatic function.

DANDELION: HOW TO USE IT FOR EPI

There are several ways to include dandelion in a pancreatic support program. Drinking dandelion tea is one typical approach. To make dandelion tea, steep the plant's dried leaves or roots in boiling water. This makes it possible to extract and eat the dandelion's beneficial components in an easily digested form. Regular ingestion of the tea can be incorporated into a comprehensive strategy for pancreatic health.

Furthermore, dandelion supplements—which come in a variety of forms, including tinctures and capsules—offer a practical means of incorporating the herb into daily routines. Before beginning any herbal supplementation, though, it is imperative to speak with a healthcare provider, particularly for people with pre-existing medical disorders or those on other prescriptions.

Dandelion shows promise for improving pancreatic health, especially when combined with EPI. It's a great herbal alternative for people looking for non-invasive ways to improve pancreatic function because of its capacity to promote digestion, lower inflammation, and supply vital nutrients. Dandelion, whether ingested as a tea or as a supplements, can contribute significantly to a comprehensive plan for pancreatic support.

MARSHMALLOW ROOT

Althaea officinalis, the scientific name for marshmallow root, is a herb that has been used traditionally in many different medical applications for a very long time. Marshmallow root has drawn attention to its possible advantages in pancreatic support. Mucilage is a gel-like material found in marshmallow root that has several benefits, one of which is that it can soothe the gastrointestinal tract.

ADVANTAGES FOR HEPATIC FUNCTION

Marshmallow root has several advantages for pancreatic health. First off, the mucilage it contains can coat the lining of the digestive system, especially the pancreas, to provide protection. Those with pancreatic problems may get relief from inflammation and discomfort thanks to this protective layer. Additionally, marshmallow root has a reputation for being able to calm and lessen inflammation, which is very advantageous for people who have pancreatic disorders.

It has been established that marshmallow root may help maintain pancreatic function, particularly in diseases such as exocrine pancreatic insufficiency (EPI). EPI is a disorder that causes problems with adequate food digestion because the pancreas is unable to create enough digestive enzymes. Because marshmallow root mucilage facilitates a more easily broken down food through the digestive tract, it may help reduce the symptoms of irritable bowel syndrome.

HOW TO APPLY EPI TO MARSHMALLOW ROOT

There are several ways to include marshmallow root in your regimen for pancreatic support. A popular technique is to make marshmallow root tea. After steeping dried marshmallow root in hot water for ten to fifteen minutes, filter the tea and enjoy. Mucilage that is released during steeping has the potential to coat the digestive tract and have a calming impact. Before using marshmallow root or any other herbal medicine in your regimen, you must speak with a healthcare provider, particularly if you are taking medication or already have a medical issue.

Herbal supplements are another way marshmallow root might help the pancreas. For people who would rather not drink it as a tea, these supplements are frequently offered as tinctures or capsules, which offer a practical alternative. Like any supplement, be sure it's compatible with your health and any ongoing therapies by following advised dosages and seeing a healthcare professional.

Marshmallow root may be advantageous for pancreatic health, especially in cases of end-stage insulinosis. Its high mucilage content, which has been shown to have calming and protecting qualities, may help to reduce inflammation and maintain normal pancreatic function. Adding marshmallow root to your regimen, whether as a tea or supplement, should be done under the supervision of a medical practitioner to make sure it is suitable for your particular set of needs.

CHAPTER SIX

MAKING FORMULAS USING HERBS

PUTTING HERBS TOGETHER FOR OPTIMAL EFFECT

Herbal formulae are made by carefully combining herbs to maximize their effectiveness in treating particular health issues. Combining herbs is an art form that draws from both modern scientific knowledge and traditional herbalism. Its goal is to combine each herb's distinct qualities for a more powerful and all-encompassing effect.

The intention is to formulate a well-rounded remedy that takes into account individual constitutions, possible interactions between herbs, and the main problem. This holistic approach recognizes the interdependence of many body systems and aims to bring balance back through the synergistic effects of carefully chosen herbs.

ADMINISTRATION & DOSAGE

For herbal formulae to be both safe and effective, dosage and administration are essential. The right dosage must be chosen after taking into account the patient's age, weight, general health, and the severity of the ailment being treated. To determine a baseline dosage, herbalists frequently refer to empirical research and historical usage; nevertheless, individual differences may call for modifications. Achieving a balance between preventing probable adverse effects and delivering a therapeutic impact is crucial. The best absorption and use of the herbal contents are facilitated by proper administration, whether the herbal ingredients are taken as teas, tinctures, capsules, or topical applications.

TRACKING DEVELOPMENT AND MODIFYING FORMULAS

A crucial component of the herbal formulation is progress monitoring, which entails tracking how each patient reacts to the suggested herbal cure. This continuous evaluation enables practitioners to determine the formula's efficacy and make any required modifications. Several factors are carefully taken into account, including any changes in symptoms, general health, and any adverse effects. To adapt formulae to changing health demands, one could change the amount, change the herbal combination, or add new herbs. Herbal formulations must be flexible and adaptive to customize therapies to the unique and changing nature of each patient's medical condition.

Regular contact between the patient and the herbalist is a vital part of the process of tracking improvement. This cooperative method makes it easier to fine-tune the herbal mix and promotes a deeper understanding of each person's experiences. Herbalists who communicate well can obtain insightful input, improve their concoctions, and decide on the best course of action for continued therapy. Given that every person reacts to herbs differently, this dynamic exchange between the practitioner and the client emphasizes the customized and holistic aspect of herbal medicine.

Developing herbal formulae is a complex process that combines scientific understanding, empirical information, and tradition. The goal of the herbal combination is to address the underlying causes of health problems and promote general well-being to maximize efficacy. The safe and efficient use of herbal treatments is ensured by dosage and administration considerations, and continuing changes to maximize therapeutic effects are made possible by progress monitoring. The skill of crafting personalized and adaptable herbal remedies that complement each patient's distinct constitution and medical history is the essence of herbal formulation art.

CHAPTER SEVEN

INCLUDING HERBAL REMEDIES IN LIFESTYLE ADJUSTMENTS

Combining lifestyle modifications with herbal therapies is a comprehensive strategy to enhance general health. Dietary guidelines are essential to this integration since what we eat has a direct impact on our health. Herbal medicines can work better when combined with a nutrient-rich, balanced diet. For example, some herbs can be used in conjunction with particular dietary patterns; for example, anti-inflammatory herbs can be used in conjunction with a diet high in fruits, vegetables, and omega-3 fatty acids to support joint health. Furthermore, when incorporating herbal medicines into one's lifestyle, it is crucial to take into account specific dietary requirements and constraints.

A healthy lifestyle includes stress reduction and exercise, which complement herbal medicines nicely. Frequent exercise not only strengthens the heart but also helps the body function more naturally, which improves the body's ability to absorb and assimilate herbal substances. The body's stress response can be comprehensively supported by combining herbal therapies with exercise, such as adaptogenic herbs with a fitness routine. The advantages of herbal medicines can be further enhanced by stress management approaches such as mindfulness and meditation, which target the underlying causes of numerous health disorders associated with stress.

A healthy lifestyle that includes things like getting enough sleep and being hydrated is crucial to optimizing the effectiveness of herbal medicines. The body's healing and regeneration processes depend on getting enough sleep, and some herbs, like chamomile or valerian, can be used to help relax and improve the quality of your sleep. Overall health depends on being hydrated and drinking herbal teas or infusions can be a tasty method to increase water intake while also reaping additional health benefits. A comprehensive approach to holistic health also includes avoiding exposure to environmental pollutants and incorporating relaxing techniques into daily routines.

Herbal medicines and lifestyle modifications work in concert to promote mental and emotional health. The impact of herbal therapies on mental health can be enhanced by establishing a sense of purpose, participating in joyful activities, and cultivating happy relationships. Incorporating adaptogenic herbal treatments, like holy basil or ashwagandha, into a lifestyle that prioritizes positive mental health practices may be very helpful in promoting emotional resilience and mood regulation.

Including herbal medicines with lifestyle modifications necessitates a comprehensive strategy that takes into account food selection, physical activity, stress reduction, and additional lifestyle elements. This holistic viewpoint emphasizes the value of individualized and long-lasting activities by acknowledging the connections between different facets of life and health.

9 798871 364895